This book is sold and/or distributed with the understanding that the publisher and author is not engaged in rendering legal or other professional services. **This book and its subject matter are for entertainment purposes only.** In this publication there may be inadvertent inaccuracies including technical inaccuracies, typographical inaccuracies and other possible inaccuracies. **The writer and publisher of this publication expressly disclaim all liability for the use or interpretation by anybody of information contained in this publication.** The author, publisher and distributors of this publication hereby disclaim any and all liability for any loss or damage caused by errors or omissions resulted from negligence, accident, or any other causes. If legal advice or other expert assistance is required, the services of a competent professional person in a consultation capacity should be sought. Products, services and websites' content vary with time. Please verify any published information.

THE PS-SPOT ORGASM: Don't Wait Any Longer For This Kind of Pleasure

By Michelle Tallia
Copyright © 2014

ISBN-13: 978-1499253597
ISBN-10: 1499253591

PS-Spot.com

First Printing

This book comes with four free bonus books (making it a $34.75 total value!) Your books are presented in this order:

Legal Notice: In this publication there may be inadvertent inaccuracies including technical inaccuracies, typographical inaccuracies and other possible inaccuracies. The writer and publisher of this publication expressly disclaim all liability for the use or interpretation by others of information contained in this publication and/or listed Web sites. The author, publisher and distributors of this publication hereby disclaim any and all liability for any loss or damage caused by errors or omissions, (should these exist) whether such errors or omissions resulted from negligence, accident, or other causes. If legal advice or other expert assistance is required, the services of a competent professional person in a consultation capacity should be sought. the information contained herein may be subject to varying state and/or local laws or regulations. All users are advised to retain competent counsel to determine what state and/or local laws or regulations may apply to the user's particular business. The Purchaser or Reader of this publication assumes responsibility for the use of these materials and information. Adherence to all applicable laws and regulations, federal, state, and local, governing professional licensing, business practices, advertising, and all other aspects of doing business in the United States or any other jurisdiction is the sole responsibility of the Purchaser or Reader. The Author and Publisher assume no responsibility or liability whatsoever on the behalf of any Purchaser or Reader of these materials. Any perceived slights of specific people or organizations are unintentional. Products, services and websites' content vary with time. Please verify any published information.

Absolutely Essential Tips For Buying & Selling On eBay

Copyright 2013

*eBay is a registered trademark of eBay Inc.

Important Tips for Buying on eBay

1) Last Minute Bidding Frenzies - Perhaps you've noticed that often there's a bidding frenzy in the last one minute of bidding. New bidders may suddenly start bidding in the hope that the previous bidders will not be watching or can't increase their bid in time. Often however it's because of *Sniping*.

Sniping websites automatically bid on your behalf, often in the last 10ish seconds. Simply sign up, enter an eBay item number and the maximum price you're willing to pay. Hidbid.com and goofbid.com offer sniping services that place bids for you.

Typically you'll need to give sniping sites your eBay password for them to work (ugh!!) Obviously that is a serious security concern.

There's little protection from eBay if things go wrong when sniping, since you willingly gave your password to a third party. If you do sign up for such a service, never use the same password for eBay as you use for other accounts like banks accounts or email addresses.

2) Second-chance Auction Scams, Beware of Them - Unscrupulous people sometimes watch bidders in high-dollar auctions and try to take unsuspecting buyer's money after an auction ends.

The scheme, known as a *Second-chance Auction Scam*, is just one of many types of Internet auction frauds reported to the *Internet Crime Complaint Center,* or *IC3.*

Second-chance scammers wait until auctions end and then offer bidders that lost, a phony second chance to purchase the item -- usually through a wire transfer service. This happens more often than people realize, beware!

3) Misspelling Search Tool - typojoe.com, goofbid.com, bargainchecker.com, fatfingers.co.uk and baycrazy.com - There are many items listed on eBay every day that have misspelled words in the title. It's unfortunate for the seller but chances are good those listings will not come up well in eBay's search engine (because misspelling causes keyword problems) and thus not bring the seller top dollar. Their loss can be your gain!

4) *Bidding Tip* - Often sellers start auctions at .99 cents, (or at least under a dollar) hoping a bidding war will erupt. Many items go unspotted, staying at this super-low price (99 cents). Software exists to hunt for eBay auctions due to finish within an hour but where the price still is low.

With these items in particular, double-check delivery charges, as some sellers hope to recoup costs by charging a little extra (though eBay's now set maximum delivery charges for many categories).

5) *Don't Forget About Facebook* - *Facebook Marketplace* is a force to be reckoned with. Also sellers often are open to haggling. Just log on to your account at Facebook and search for "Marketplace". It's also worth checking to see if there's any local Facebook selling groups in your area.

6) *Nigerian Type Scam for Paying*. These unscrupulous people want to pay with a money order that they claim to already have handy. Often it's for more than the purchase amount. He writes to ask if the seller would be "honest enough" (or something of that nature) to send him the extra cash along with the item. (However he might just try to only buy the item with it and not ask for extra cash.) Unfortunately the money order can look okay but is counterfeit. They particularly like the *Buy It Now* feature.

7) *Set Long-term Alerts For Rare Items* - If you want something very specific or hard to find, set a 'favorite search' and eBay will email each time a seller lists your desired item.

Simply type a product in eBay's search bar, such as "silver dollar", and click 'save search'. Be as specific as possible for the most accurate results. When (and if) someone lists one, you're alerted with an email.

8) Don't Assume eBay's the Cheapest Place To Get Your Item - Many people assume that if it's on eBay, it's automatically the least expensive place to get it, but that often isn't the case. Perhaps you'd also like to use *shopbots* (shopping robots) that check numerous Internet retailers to find the best price. Type into a search engine "shopping comparison sites".

The same rule applies when buying used merchandise. Check used marketplaces on <u>Amazon.com</u> and <u>craigslist.com</u> - you may even get it for free on <u>Freecycle.com</u> or <u>Freegle.com</u>.

9) Check the eBay Going Rate For an Item - There's a quick way to check an eBay product's average price. Enter the item into the search box and click "completed listings". What will come up is a list of prices that similar auctions have already settled on. After that, sort it by "Price: lowest first". If the price is red, it means no one bought it. Green means it sold. Figure out the average price.

10) eBay has banned the selling of intangible items, and that includes curses! - Among the items that were prohibited as of August 30, 2012, are "advice; spells; curses; hexing; conjuring; magic; prayers; blessing services; magic potions; healing sessions; work from home businesses and information; wholesale lists, and drop shop lists."

11) Haggling on eBay Can Pay Off - There's nothing wrong with asking for a discount, even if the listing doesn't have the "make offer" indication. Haggling works best on *Buy It Now* listings, or auctions with a high start price and no bids. Also you'll likely do better if you haggle as the auction is coming closer to closing as the seller could start feeling more desperate.

To contact the seller, click on the seller's nickname then "ask seller a question". If you're polite, you'll likely get further. Blunt requests such as "dude, how about $15?" likely won't work out as well. Remember the seller is likely going to lose money doing this so no point in being annoying.

Once you've arranged a deal, try to keep the transaction within eBay. Ask the seller to add (or change) a Buy It Now price. That way you don't lose the usual eBay buyer protection privileges.

12) Other Things to Do To Exploit Sellers' Screw-ups - Some sellers make basic mistakes, leavings goods going for bargain money.

As well as spelling boo-boos, another error is to leave out key details such as shoe size, dress brand, saying a console's an a Wii when the photo shows a Xbox. At this point, many buyers give it up as "too much hassle".

So contact the seller to fill in gaps, but don't ask the question via the item's listing page, (because that way, when the seller replies, eBay lets them add their reply to the main listing, so it's no longer your secret.)

Instead, ask the question via the seller's profile (make it clear which item you're talking about). They might not bother with the extra hassle of adding it to the listing, so you'll be the only one in the know.

Also the seller might not realize how pricy an item he/she actually has.

13) Tool to Track Down Crazy End Times - Listings that finish at anti-social times often get fewer bids, thus sell for less. To locate auctions that finish when fewer people are around to bid on them, use BayCrazy's *Crazy End Time* search. (A lot more on the best times to end your auction in the next section of the book "*Selling on eBay*".)

Check out their auto-bidding tools if you don't want to spend all that time in front of the computer bidding at odd times. Other BayCrazy.com tools include "unwanted gift" and "ending now" searches.   www.baycrazy.com/search.php?page=nightowl (Baycrazy offers other eBay related opportunities also.)

14) Search Descriptions as Well as Titles - eBay automatically searches seller's titles for results that include your specified keywords. If you're not getting the results you want, try also searching the item's *description* too. (To do this go to Advanced Search.)

For example, imagine you were searching for a REI Jacket. Unfortunately the seller may be selling one but only put "Ski Jacket" in the title however he mentioned "REI" in the description. Include description in your search and then it should then come up.

15) Search Using eBay Boolean Logic - If a seller could describe an item different ways, you can make eBay search for several different ways of describing it at once. Just enter different phrases individually enclosed by quotation marks or "( )", then followed by commas.

So for example, type... "fishing tackle", "hook", "reel" ...and it will simultaneously bring up listings that contain the words "fishing tackle", "hook" and/or "reel".

16) Add A Few Extra Cents to Your Bid - When bidding, you enter a "maximum bid", and eBay makes automatic bids on your behalf up to your maximum bid.

Don't enter a round number. For example, if a coat is currently selling for $20, and the most you are willing to pay for it is $25, enter a maximum bid of $25.24. If someone tries to outbid you by entering the round number of $25, they will receive an outbid notice. eBay will go your bid, even though it's just 24 cents more.

17) Be Somewhat Skeptical of Feedback - eBay sellers have a feedback rating that acts as a useful guide to previous seller's opinion's of them. As a guideline, look for a seller with more than 98% positive feedback and a high feedback score of at least 30. Also ensure you read their feedback from their *selling*, not just their *buying*. (To see their feedback, click on their username).

18) Seller with Zero Feedback Could be Cause For Concern - Think twice before purchasing expensive items from a seller with zero feedback.

Remember feedback's useful but not infallible. One thing to watch for is traders selling a number of cheap things for $1ish each to build their feedback, and suddenly listing items costing hundreds each.

19) Check to Make Sure You're Bidding on the Actual Item - Sometimes you assume you're bidding for an item on eBay (or any auction site,) when all that's actually being sold is a link to another site selling it. People are not suppose to be able to sell these on eBay but they can fall through the cracks.

Always read the whole description in detail before bidding. Often the catch is hidden in the text at the end – an attempt to protect the seller from any recourse.

20) Scam - Beware of it - It's a red flag if a seller writes "Before bidding, contact me" then asks for a money transfer. Thieves who hijack actual eBay accounts might use this tactic.

21) Scam - Beware of it - Always be worried if you're asked to pay by an instant money transfer service such as Western Union or MoneyGram. Instant money transfer payments cannot be traced and are highly popular with thieves.

22) Sneakily Find Underpriced Buy It Nows - Feel free to hunt for Buy It Now bargains also. Perhaps the seller under-values their item making their price a good deal.

These steals are snapped up quickly. Go to "Advanced Search", select a category you're interested in, filter it to show *Buy It Now* items and sort the results.

23) Always Complain within 30-45 Days - Under eBay's buyer protection program, 30-45 days is the most number of days you have to open a case if you're unhappy with your purchase. (There are some exceptions such as tickets for events that are months away.) Read more on eBay's protection policy. http://pages.ebay.com/coverage/index.html

Under eBay's own Buyer Protection rules, buyers are eligible for a refund if the item's "not as described", meaning it didn't match the seller's description. http://pages.ebay.com/coverage/index.html

24) Pay by PayPal - Avoid sending checks and never use money orders. It's much harder for scammers to disappear with your cash when you use eBay's online payment system, PayPal.

Paying this way costs the same as paying by check, but means you're covered by eBay's Buyer Protection program. If an item is faulty, counterfeit or non-existent, you are far more likely to get a refund.

25) Outbid? Don't Give Up On It Yet - Missed out on a desired item by pennies? Don't give up hope. As every seller knows, sales sometimes don't materialize when buyers change their minds or can't come up with the dough. Because of that feel free to send a friendly message such as: "Hi, I've been looking for this poster for years and just saw your finished auction. Please let me know if the sale doesn't come through."

They may send a *Second-chance Offer*, which are sent out by sellers to unsuccessful bidders if the winner fails to pay up. Ask them to relist at an agreed *Buy It Now* price.

26) Know Your Consumer Rights - When buying from a person who makes or sells goods for resale on eBay you often have the same rights as when buying in person from a shop that does the same. This means your goods must be of satisfactory quality and as described.

With private sellers it's buyer beware. Buyers' only rights under law are that the product is fairly described and the owner has the right to sell it.

Under eBay's own Buyer Protection rules, buyers are eligible for a refund if the item is "not as described", meaning it doesn't match the seller's description.

27) Beware of All The Fakes - While eBay has a 'flag and remove' policy to help identify fakes, still plenty fall through the cracks.

If you're buying big-name brands, do your research first. Carefully check sellers' feedback and post on the forum's eBay board to get others' opinions. Be especially wary of overseas sellers or branded items that seem especially cheap.

The more *unprofessional* the photos, likely the better. Thieves often take professional photos from the brands' sites. Legitimate sellers typically take photos of items at home that might not come out as well.

28) Think Twice Before You Give A Seller Negative Feedback - Of course, negative feedback is often justified but have a heart, don't leave negative or even *neutral* feedback without first trying to work the issue out with the seller. Most sellers are good folks who will try to help particularly, as it can mean a lot to their business to stay in your good graces.

Remember eBay users can view the feedback you've left for others, and if you leave a significant amount of negative feedback, they may well decide you're too high of a risk to sell to.

29) Add An Item You're Interested in to eBay's "Watch List" - Want to keep track of an item without bidding on it? eBay lets you add items to a "Watch List", so you can relax knowing you'll get an email reminder within 36 hours of the auction ending. To watch an item, just click the *"add to watch list"* link in the upper part of the item's eBay webpage.

30) Don't Do Private Purchasing - Sellers may suggest you do a deal outside eBay for a cheaper price. If you do you'll likely have less protection if things go bad. You won't be able to leave negative feedback and you won't be protected by eBay's Buyer Protection Plan.

31) Think Safety When Picking Up An Item In Person - The usual precautions apply. If you get to their door and the seller's holding a butcher knife, now's the time to run.

32) Think International - There's bargains to be had on overseas eBay sites. To include foreign auctions in search results, click "worldwide" for location.

Still can't find what you want? Another option is buying directly from *international* eBay sites. The main ones are USA, Canada, Australia, Germany, France and Spain - there's a full list at the bottom of eBay's homepage. Make sure that the item reads "Shipping to: *worldwide*" before bidding as some international sellers only do business with their country's buyers.

Always factor in postage and if applicable, custom fees. Remember that return postage fees could be hefty.

Also what kind of credit card protections will there be? You're often still protected by eBay and PayPal's buyer protections (if you use PayPal), but it's worth investigating. Type in "buyer protection" in PayPal.

33) Don't Forget The Online Classified Ads - Again, let's not assume that because it's on eBay, that's where you'll get the best price for an item. Unfortunately that's often just not the case. Type "top classified ad sites" or something of that nature, into search engines. There's also *Freecycle* and *Freegle*. (Those two sites offer free stuff. freecycle.org and ilovefreegle.org.)

Remember, anyone can post on these classified ad sites. If someone asks you to pay by MoneyGram or Western Union, as always be concerned. It's a bad way to pay.

34) Check Other Auction Sites Also - There are other auction sites that can be found through search engines. If you're searching for something specific, it's also worth adding it to your search. *Auctionlotwatch*.com is a useful shopbot for online auctions. Search for an item and it trawls the big auction sites for you.

35) Check Cashback and Voucher Websites - Check cashback websites to see if there's money back available on your eBay purchase. Type into search engines: "cashback and voucher sites".

Cashback sites give you a cut of their proceeds by setting you up with product and/or service providers.

36) eBay has trained teachers that could be in your area. Also see eBay University. Check out:
http://pages.ebay.com/sellerinformation/howtosell/university.html

Important Tips for Selling on eBay

1) Join eBay Forums - Ask questions about anything, selling, buying etc. Great information is posted already and could be of use. Work together as a team. Find eBay and other auction forums by looking those up in search engines. Ebay has forums also. http://forums.ebay.com/category/Ebay-Discussion-Boards/2001

2) eBay Research Tool 1 - To help in your research about selling items, you can go Type into a search engine "best selling eBay items." EBay provides that information.

3) eBay Research Tool 2 - You can use Ebuyers (www.ebuyersedge.com) to just search eBay for items as well as set up a saved eBay search (or a number of them). You'll get alerted with an e-mail when a matching item is listed.

4) Second-chance Offers - If the buyer of your item falls through, you can send the other bidders a *Second-chance Offer* to see if they're still interested in buying it.

5) Keywords & Relevancy - Make sure the brand name of what you're selling is in the title! If you're selling a Champion Portable Generator, your listing title should include the make and model number, in this case "New Champion 42431 Portable Generator, 1500 Watt". Your listing title should be a short, abbreviated description of the item you are selling.

The name of the product in the title has to do with the search results (keywords). If people want to buy your portable generator they may search "portable generator, generator, Champion, Champion portable generator," etc. You want to make your listing show up in as many search results as possible.

In review, a wild but catchy title will definitely grab the attention of most people who see it, but won't come up in many people's search results, unless also in the title listing is the name of the product that people would type in when looking for it. (Even that's not guaranteed to work.)

6) If a potential customer wants other people's opinions on a product you sell, you might want to send them to the Amazon.com's webpage for the site as Amazon posts feedback from buyers of that same product. Make sure that Amazon is not selling it for less than you are or that idea could backfire!

7) *Mention Flaws*: If there is a flaw in the item you are selling, make sure you mention it (though try to call it something else like "scratch" or "mark" if that's what it is.) If your product has a flaw and you don't mention it in your listing, you could get negative feedback and a request for a refund from the person who buys the "flawed" item.

If possible, make the flaw sound positive. You could say "this product has a small dent that has no effects on its operation, but because of this you save big bucks!"

Mentioning a flaw also can make you look like an honest person. You can even have the flaw mentioned in your bullet points - Small scratch on the top (saves you money!!)

8) *Host Your Own Pictures* - You can host your own pictures on another website or your eBay Store and thus show many, many more photos free of charge.

9) *Payment Options:* - You should offer the customer several different choices of payment. Most of your customers will pay you through PayPal, (PayPal is owned by eBay,) so make sure you get a PayPal account (www.paypal.com). Of course, not everyone who buys items on eBay prefers PayPal, some may prefer Western union's Bidpay or another payment system.

Wire Transfers - Unscrupulous overseas buyers prefer these as they're not as traceable. It's preferable not to take them.

10) *Offering SquareTrade Warranties* - If applicable to what you're selling, another good way to build trust is to sign up for SquareTrade warranties at www.squaretrade.com. www.squaretrade.com/seller-faq

11) About Me Page - The About Me page is often overlooked by many eBay sellers (and buyers.) While having the free About Me page likely will not dramatically increase your sales, it can help if you have good things to say about yourself and a nice picture. Note, many sellers only include links to their listings and maybe not enough information about themselves in the About Me page.

12) People Bidding with 0 Feedback ratings - Having a good to great feedback rating is so important as you know. Many sellers refuse letting members with 0 feedback bid on their auctions. Getting a negative feedback from somebody that unpredictable is simply a risk we don't want to take. In many cases, we simply don't trust them.

13) Best Time To End Your Auction - The best time for an auction to close (end) is in the evenings and on weekends as that's when most people are on the Internet for that type of activity! You want to make sure that when your auction is closing (ending), everyone that's interested in it is available to bid on it. The mornings are the times that the eBay website gets the least visitors (as people are more often sleeping or working.)

If you live in the Eastern Time Zone, list your auction between 9pm-11pm, Central Time Zone list between 8-10pm, Mountain Time Zone between 7-9pm, and for the Pacific Time Zone list between 6-8pm. This will give you the biggest exposure at the end of your auction. The debate is out as to what day your auction should end on. Some sellers report that Tuesday, Wednesday and Thursday are best. Other sellers report that Saturday and Sunday are best.

There are a few exceptions though. For example, some business products sell best during weekdays and during work hours. Obviously this is because people are usually ordering those types of products at work, for work. Studies have shown that a listing that ends at peak hours can attract up to 25% more bids than one that ends in non-peak hours. Listing your auctions at optimal times is one of the easiest ways to attract more bids.

To end the auction in the evenings, you'll need to put the item for sale in the evening (*or use listing software [see next page] to do it for you*) as eBay considers each day to have a length of 24 hours.

Note, it's eBay's practice that when someone's auction is ending, that listing shows up higher on keyword search results (which is a good thing!)

14) Terms of Service Webpage (Yours) - That's something even a lot of experienced sellers don't seem to include, though it likely won't be necessary if all the information is already in your FAQ webpage. For instance, what's the return policy? What are the shipping options, and what will they cost? What are the accepted methods of payment? How soon is payment to be sent? What is the warranty?

15) Listing Software (For Your Items) - Listing software organizes your eBay listings making the listing part of your business simpler and more efficient. There are many different kinds of listing software. You can do an Internet search for them.

Turbo Lister is free software from eBay. Turbo Lister allows you to upload thousands of listings at a time. It saves listings, schedules your listings and uploads them to eBay automatically. Using it you can edit multiple listings at the same time, preview what your listings will look like before uploading them and more. More eBay software is offered at:
     http://pages.ebay.com/help/sell/advanced_selling_tools.html

16) Drop Shipping What You Sell - With drop shipping all you have to do is list items up for auction and when they sell, you contact your supplier, who ships the products from their factory, straight to your customers. In theory drop shipping is a good way to go, but it could offer problems. What happens when you sell items and your supplier sends them to the wrong addresses? What happens when you sell items and your supplier is out of stock? In those cases your reputation suffers. If you are going to use drop shipping; make sure there is good communication between you and your supplier (drop shipper.) Also make sure you have some products in stock in case the supplier runs out by the time your auctions have closed.

17) eBay Stores - eBay stores can be great if you have a number of items to sell. First you'll need to reach the minimum number of feedbacks required (10) to open one. Most PowerSellers have eBay stores. Store sellers can see an increase in profit of up to 25% in the first three months of opening the store (according to eBay). Having your own eBay store can save you a substantial amount of money in listing fees and let you sell items in a fixed price format as well as selling via auctions. Also you can list items for a much longer time and store them in your inventory list for 30, 60, 90, 120 days and even "Good till Cancelled". You can feature links to other auctions in all your listings by utilizing a cross promotion tool. There are also bonuses like your own search engine and monthly reports from eBay featuring statistics and dada about your sales in the past month.

An eBay store also gives you a location. It gives you a base of operation, a place where people can easily find you, and a place where repeat customers can come back to. Your customers will be able to bookmark and return to your store, and it may also be indexed in the major search engines. So if you're selling silver dollars, and someone does a BING search for silver dollars, your eBay store may appear in the results along with the usual online retail websites! Obviously this can increase your traffic greatly, and likewise boost your sales.

18) Your eBay Store Identity - Ideally your eBay store should look different from your competition. You can use the design templates eBay offer you, but perhaps it's best to use original graphics. Fortunately eBay Stores are customizable. Ideally, to establish your name, your eBay store should appear like your listings as much as possible. Same colors, design and look.

19) Get a Domain Name - You need to get a simple and memorable domain name. A domain name makes it simple for people to find you. The standard web address eBay will give to your store will look like this: *stores.ebay.com/yourname*, this is not a very memorable web address and it's too long to be easy to type into a web browser. It would be best if you had a web address like *mystore.com*.

The End

This book is sold and/or distributed with the understanding that the publisher and author is not engaged in rendering legal or other professional services. **This book and its subject matter are for entertainment purposes only.** In this publication there may be inadvertent inaccuracies including technical inaccuracies, typographical inaccuracies and other possible inaccuracies. **The writer and publisher of this publication expressly disclaim all liability for the use or interpretation by anybody of information contained in this publication.** The author, publisher and distributors of this publication hereby disclaim any and all liability for any loss or damage caused by errors or omissions resulted from negligence, accident, or any other causes. If legal advice or other expert assistance is required, the services of a competent professional person in a consultation capacity should be sought. Products, services and websites' content vary with time. Please verify any published information.

Book #2 - 100 Good Line to Put in Your Personal Ad

100 Good Lines To Put in Your Personal Ad

Introduction

The lines in this book can be combined with other lines you may think of to make your personal ad all it can be. Some lines in the book might need adapting to best suit you.

TAGLINES: Your short "tagline" is a headline that, perhaps along with your picture, can get readers to further explore your ad. Great taglines are like gold and people have paid hundreds of dollars for them! Now however many are on the Internet for you to see and use.

Remember, people love to laugh. A funny tagline is a big plus.

There is a great deal of material in this book to build quality taglines from. You may also want to take a bit of time and do a web search for "best personal ad taglines" for ideas. Chances are others (including those looking at your ad) haven't seen the tagline already, or have forgotten it if they did.

The Lines

A day not in love is a lost opportunity.

My friends know me as spontaneous, spritely, and upbeat.

I am searching for a beautiful person inside and out.

Are you looking for real love and someone special?

I enjoy thought provoking dialogue.

Together let's seek our destiny.

I hope only to fulfill your every desire. Is that too much to ask?

I love making people happy and to see them smile, even if at times it is at my own expense.

I feel the most pleasure when I know I am doing/enduring something to please another.

I'm looking to learn, not just to play....

I'd like to explore hidden fantasies with you.

I want to be taken to that special place and beyond.

I have the financial and emotional capacity to take care of myself.

Unlike perhaps others here I'm not misrepresenting myself. I know the importance of honesty.

I love sex. Rough sex, fun sex, emotional sex... I want you to respect me before and after but during is negotiable.

I want to explore my naughty side.

I'm looking for a friend, confidant and lover.

Like me I'd like you to be thoughtful, attractive, and looking to expand yourself as a person.

I have developed intricate pleasure techniques which can slowly arouse and pleasure beyond imagination.

I think I would describe myself, briefly, as quite a sociable person with a good sense of humor who doesn't take herself too seriously...having said that I believe I am also thoughtful and caring and someone who places great value on good friendships and relationships.

I am loyal, compassionate and respectful of people and animals. People describe me as easy going and good natured.

I have got great plans and goals in my life which I want to achieve.

I'm a contemporary yet spiritual soul in search of his charming, compassionate and caring companion to share this journey of life.

Are you looking for someone to grow with and push things further?

I have a wise mind and younger spirit.

I am an easy going, and loyal friend.

I'm looking forward to a fantastic voyage of a relationship.

I am attracted to someone who enjoys learning and growing.

Are you looking for fun, adventure and a challenge? If so I'm your girl.

I'm a passionate person with interests numerous and diverse.

I am trustworthy, affectionate, passionate, loving and non-judgmental. I am happy with myself and my accomplishments.

I want someone kind, loving, honest, communicative and self-aware. Your developed interest in education, hygiene, aesthetics, style and emotional literacy would make life easier for us. I'd like to find someone interested in building a relationship based on an accomplished life and a win/win attitude.

I am looking for someone who can work themselves deep inside my mind and make me fall to my knees.

Are you looking for someone to make you happy...someone that won't just have sex with you but will make love to you?

We all want to achieve heart pounding serenity.

I am looking for something more than just sex and games. Sure sex is a part of it but I also want someone that I can spend time with. I want the total package.

I want someone that I can go out with, talk with, laugh with, and fall in love with.

Outside of our playtime, I'd like to enjoy a harmony that can grow into a loving, trusting relationship. I enjoy the outdoors and staying healthy, going out on the town from time to time and hanging out at home.

My last relationship ended because we grew in different directions.

I am usually lucky and love life. I would like to find someone like that.

I'm a strong, seductive, passionate woman who is established and knows herself.

I'm well educated and well-travelled. I'm gainfully employed and very independent. I enjoy traveling, good food and wine, the theater and sports.

I'm searching for an open minded man with an adventurous soul and sensual heart. A journey in love is the destination. We still have plenty of time but none to waste! A beautiful world is waiting. Let's enjoy while we can!

I'll laugh at your corny jokes.

I'm a writer and voracious reader. I'm smart, and I like smart people.

Physical attraction leads to animal instincts.

I have a strong passion for the exploration and power of touch in all its forms.

I enjoy knowledge, I like to learn new and exciting things.

I am cosmopolitan and highly educated. I am a baby boomer, in good shape and would like an agemate and a partner who understands mutuality.

I am interested in developing a long term relationship.

I am interested in meeting someone who is honest, open and enjoys (his) her kink.

I have very many interests and I'm passionate about all of them! I love movies, literature, music, art, theatre, science... and lots of other things.

I am fun, open-minded, spontaneous and down for raunchy action.

The reason openness is important to me is that it shows that someone accepts themselves.

I'm lively and active and have a well developed sense of humor.

I hope to always be me and take advantage of any opportunities and chances whenever they're thrown at me.

I am totally devoted when in love.

I'm a laid-back, drama-free kind of person.

I want to be late to my own funeral.

Physical play is quite enjoyable but chemistry and a connection is more important.

I like to laugh, I like to have fun.

I believe that love is not what we see but what we do.

I won't ignore you or abandon you. I'm not looking for a secondary relationship.

I have a well developed and dominant sexual identity. I am seeking a man who is a smart, uninhibited, challenging partner.

I consider myself a natural leader, an innovator, a creator. I fight for the best and readily take the risks incumbent with leading a fulfilled, enriched life.

I am a strong, confident thinker, with a secure sense of himself (herself).

I consider myself to be a spontaneous, fun loving person. I work hard, play hard, and enjoy life. I'm a very affectionate and passionate. I like to hold hands and believe it or not cuddle. I believe in treating others the way I would like to be treated. I am looking for someone to grow with spiritually, mentally and physically. I want someone who is not afraid to love and be loved, someone who is affectionate, passionate and good kisser.

I will love you and take good care of you. I am someone who you can trust and believe in, someone who will always want to make you feel happy.

I'm neat and clean both internally and externally.

I want true love and real commitment.

I am looking for something more than just sex and games. There is a balance that is needed since none of us can live in a purely sexual world. Sure sex is an important part of it all but I also want someone that I can spend time with. I want the total package. I want someone I can go out with, talk with, laugh with, and fall in love with.

I want something that will naturally grow and evolve into its own very beautiful story.

I enjoy a great number of things and am very open to experimentation.

I'm interested in your fantasies.

I want to touch your body, your soul, your life.

I still believe that fairytales can come true, it can happen to us...
I live a healthy lifestyle. I am seeking the same.

I am brimming with sexual desire.

I will be looking forward to hear from you and Your wish will always be done...

I am looking for a partner - but I am happy to form a friendship.

Living on earth is expensive...but it does include free trips around the sun.

I eat healthy and workout regularly.

I am an educated, intelligent professional with eclectic tastes in most everything: art, music, food, people, entertainment and travel.

I'm looking for a non-smoker to share my life with in all ways, a friend and companion to travel with, commiserate over bad days and rejoice over good days; a lover and confidant.

Educated, professional and kinky.

I have class and style. I know the value of dressing to impress.

I would love to be able to say "I've finally found you."

I believe that we all have the ability to create or change anything.

I consider myself to be a sharp, crafty, inventive, fun, strong woman who enjoys life more when she's in a relationship.

I'm looking for a like minded man to chat, debate and play with.

I'm not a just fantasist wasting your time.

I am people biased not gender biased.

I am family-oriented and have family values.

I possess confidence but take pride in not being arrogant. I'm persistent but respectful. I have intelligence and charm.

I don't like negative people. We're here to live life not fear it.

I have learned in life that the smallest good deed is better than the grandest good intention.

I have high hopes for us.

I am a sharp, crafty, inventive, fun woman who doesn't hate men or hate anyone for that matter.

I enjoy life so much more when I'm in a relationship.

What you are like OUT of bed makes you more desirable for me to want you to take me there.

I like to please as much as be pleased.

I want to discover and explore my limits as well as push them further.

I like intellectual conversations.

My ambition is self-actualisation, to release the potential within.

I'm thoughtful, devoted, industrious, competitive, genuine and trustworthy.

I'm looking to learn and grow, not just to play....

The End

Book #3 - Breast Massage Secrets Revealed

Michelle Tallia

Copyright (C) 2014

PS-Spot.com

Breast Massage Secrets Revealed

The specialized breast massage discussed in this book can give a woman a surprising amount of pleasure. If her lover is unavailable to pleasure her this way, women can easily give themselves *Extreme Pleasure Breast Massage*, and it's something women can do to themselves for the rest of their lives.

There are a many positions a woman's body can be in to receive this specialized and very sexually arousing breast massage. For this example though, let's have her sitting up and at least topless. Do note however that as she gets more and more aroused, she'd probably prefer to be naked so one or both of you can access her pubic area with fingers or toys while she's experiencing Extreme Pleasure Breast Massage.

For this position the massager sits behind her with his/her chest up against her back. If it's okay with who is getting the massage, I suggest the massager be naked as many women will lose control at some point when getting Extreme Pleasure Breast Massage and be anxiously reaching behind their lower backs to play with the massager's privates. If a woman has never experienced this type of erotic massage before, she in particular may react with callous abandon.

Before placing yourselves in any of the massage positions, you'll need to have readily available a good supply of quality lotion, massage oil or hair conditioner (yes the stuff you might put on your hair. Thicker hair conditioner is often better and the cheaper brands might work just as well.)

If using lotion, try to use some brand of non-desensitizing lotion. (Most lotion's ingredients include desensitizers to dull the pain of dry skin and other irritations. These desensitizers can at least partially desensitize breasts, thus cutting down on the breast's capacity to provide pleasure.) Baby lotions at dollar stores may be good ones to try but lotions tend to vary by brand. Optimally you want the massaging medium to stay slippery as long as possible and, not cause any irritation of course. Cold lotion/oil/conditioner on breasts can provide an unwelcome jolt so if warming is necessary, warm the lotion/oil/conditioner up ahead of time using the microwave oven, or by setting it in hot water. Make sure the top is loosened somewhat incase it warms up too much and creates steam. (You can also rub together blobs of it in your hands to warm it up.) Always have an ample amount of this massage oil/lotion/hair conditioner nearby as well as small towels to wipe it off of your hands and her breasts after the massage is over.

Put a sizeable glob of massage oil/lotion/conditioner on each of your hands, rubbing it all over the palms of your hands to spread it out, as well as warm it if it's not yet warm. Then put your well lubricated hands on her breasts, *but not yet on her nipples and areolas*. This is because those provide the most pleasure and thus the best is saved for last!

It is so important that the massager make sure to keep his/her massaging hands *very* well lubricated. When the oil, lotion or hair conditioner is breaking down the massager will feel stickiness developing. **It is now time to put more massage oil/lotion/conditioner on!** The rule of thumb is that you can't lubricate your hands and her breasts too much!

Also the massager needs to make sure his/her nails and skin of their hands are smooth. Trim and file your fingernails and that kind of thing, to as short and smooth as possible. Otherwise she (the person receiving the massage) might feel them as they rub against her sensitive skin. She can even get hurt by them because as she is in the thongs of ecstasy, she might not realize that they are hurting her, so make sure to watch out for her and take care of this situation.

Typically the massage will provide three levels of pleasure. Massaging the fleshy part of her breast (but not massaging her areolas and nipples) should give her pronounced and very welcome pleasure; of course the faster her breasts are massaged the more pleasure she'll get.

Including her areolas in the massaging will increase her pleasure a lot. But massaging her nipples will really get her going.

Below (and not in order of importance) are suggestions on how to optimize the breast massage.

* Start from the bottom of her breasts (where the breasts meet her torso) and work your way slowly higher up to just below her areolas. You can move your hands at varying speeds but typically the faster you massage the more pleasure she'll get.

* Simultaneously circle her boobs with each hand. Start out by using limited pressure on the breasts while utilizing only one finger, then gradually work your way up to utilizing all your fingers. Go clockwise then counterclockwise (or vice-versa.) Remember, *leave her nipples and areolas alone as much as possible until she's practically (or literally) begging for you to massage them*. Sure you will "bump" into them from time to time as you massage around them. Those bumps will give her a delicious taste of what's to come.

* At its base, wrap each hand around a single breast then run your well lubricated hands around and along that breast in a steady spiraling motion up the breasts in the direction of her nipples, until you reach the edge of her areolas. Of course you can go in the opposite direction also (starting from just below her areolas and working your way down to where her boobs meets her torso.)

* Place one hand on the base of one breast; the back of the hand should be facing her head. Put your other hand on the base of her *other* breast, the back of it should be facing her legs. Slide your well lubricated hands from left to right and then vice-versa, across and along both breasts.

* At its base, take each breast in a well lubricated hand and with increasing speed pull up from the base of her breast toward the nipple until your fingers reach the edge of the areolas (or if you're already playing with her areolas and/or nipples, go all the way to her nipples.) Then do the opposite and slide your hands back down from the top of her breasts to the breast's base (where you started from.) Repeat this procedure many, many times.

* Tease her by sliding only your well lubricated, manicured fingertips over her breasts, wiggling your fingers.

* Instead of the above, perhaps for a minute or more, you'd like to start the festivities by teasing her breasts by only briefly touching them here and there using only the tips of your fingers.

* Concentrate your efforts on only one well lubricated breast; wrap both hands around it, kneading it, pulling it and twisting it.

As previously discussed, it's strongly suggested that you take your time before playing with her areolas and then nipples. This is because she will still get a good deal of pleasure from having the 'areola and nipple-less' massage. I for one require that she even beg you to play with her nipples--because as we know this is where the breasts offer the most pleasure.

Before finally massaging her nipples (admittedly you will "bump" into them periodically,) I would suggest waiting until she is already well stimulated. You may stroke her anticipation by whispering in her ear that you're about to play with her nipples, then suddenly do it! She may scream with delight as an orgasm overcomes her.

Playing with her nipples is typically the high point of the massage. She'll likely be getting the most pleasure now. (Again, the faster your well-lubricated fingers move around her nipples, the more pleasure she's likely to get.)

Okay massagers you now have a choice, you can immediately start massaging her nipples fast and hard, driving her crazy, or start massaging them slowly, then progressively massaging them faster and faster until she screams in ecstasy. If you're going to massage them fast immediately, as is the first option, many women will start their orgasm then (if they haven't already.)

Don't forget you can let her use a vibrator on herself as you massage her and thus it's suggested you keep a vibrator within her arm's reach. Believe me she'll find it if it's there.

Because so often the woman you're massaging will get so aroused from all this, that with both hands she'll instinctively reach around her lower back to play with the massager's pubic area. She then will not have a free hand to use the vibrator on herself. (Of course both your hands are busy giving her Extreme Pleasure Breast Massage.) A way to counter this is to secure a vibrator with white medical tape (the type used to hold gauge and cotton to cuts etc.) over her most sexually sensitive pubic area. (Perhaps it would be helpful if she keeps her panties on for extra support.) If you do this, more women will orgasm while you are giving her Extreme Pleasure Breast Massage.

Remember guys her nipples can get tender after orgasm and need to be left alone for at least a bit of time.

As is obvious, ladies, you can give yourself Extreme Pleasure Breast Massage in the privacy of your own bedroom.

After the massage, ladies your breasts tend to become firmer for a while and often they'll feel quite good for hours.

The following is another way of giving this massage, (told from the perspective of the kinky dominant massager.)

I will tell you to stand up and we will go to the bed (if we're not already there.) I will set the bed up so I am sitting with my back against the headboard of the bed and you are laying in front of me face-down on cushions (on the bed) with your head positioned so you can easily suck on my penis and play with my scrotum.

Also I'll put a roughly 3' x 3' sheet of plastic under your upper body to keep the massage lotion/oil/hair conditioner from going on the bed covers.

Perhaps I will also tie your hands together and perhaps then also to the headboard. If I do that though I will make sure there is enough slack in the rope for your hands to still move freely around my penis and scrotum while you suck. If your hands are tied to the headboard, I will be sitting on the rope as my butt will be in-between your bound hands and the headboard which your hands are tied to.

Your breasts will now be positioned, thanks to these cushions, just above the ground. As you suck on my penis, I will generously lubricate (and keep lubricated,) your breasts with some brand of preferably non-desensitizing massaging medium. I will warm the lotion/oil/hair conditioner up ahead of time or rub it in my hands to warm it up, if warming is necessary. I will then massage your breasts. (Many lotions put desensitizers in them to dull the pain of dry skin. These can at least partially desensitize breasts thus cutting down on the breast's capacity to provide pleasure.) I will continue for a long time to massage your lubricated breasts as you suck on my penis. (Remember to always keep the massager's hands well lubricated! The two of you will quickly notice that the nipples respond with the most pleasure from this massage.)

Using a yardstick type implement, I can reach across your back and spank you as you suck. Obviously one should make sure the woman can handle being spanked while sucking. Most can, depending on the intensity of the spanking and how hard she's already orgasming.

The End

Book #4 - Special Things To Do During 3 Hours of Sex; A Step-by-step Guide

Please note that the following sexual experience has kinky overtones to it. If you find any of that disconcerting, please use alternative aspects of this sex scene. This is written from a male dominant perspective.

Just a quick bit of information about my lovemaking style, I am a sexually dominant, heterosexual male. I need my lady love to be able to orgasm-on-demand, or agree to be trained for it. Typically she's trained to have extremely long orgasms versus several comparatively shorter ones. This is part of where my sexual dominance comes in. My lover will need to start her orgasm quickly, and continue it for as long as I am sexually stimulating her by using my hands or other parts of my body. Fortunately the human female body is built to have long, frequent and powerful orgasms, though so comparatively few women get to enjoy their incredible built-in capacity for pleasure. The truth is that orgasm-on-demand is a remarkably easy thing for women to do once properly trained.

Most men concentrate on a woman's body to stimulate her sexually, (which in and of itself is not a bad idea) but in so many cases that's not enough. I have found that most men do not adequately sexually stimulate their women's minds.

There is a natural tendency by women to be the more submissive sex during sexual activity, and that would certainly be required for the 3 hour playtime we're discussing. (Please note that if this tendency toward submissive behavior is not true in your case then this type of orgasm on demand training likely won't work too well with you.)

In her now sexually aroused state, it's normal for her subconscious mind to be more susceptible to suggestions regarding sex. People like me take it a step further and require her to do more than that during her sexual submission, specifically she will be required to orgasm long and hard, no ifs, ands or butts. Thus it is no longer her decision on how hard and long to orgasm but her lover's and I for one will require her to orgasm relentlessly.

Another way to look at it is that after being trained for orgasm on demand, the woman no longer is the one making the decision as to when she is going to have her orgasms and/or how intense the orgasm will be. She has yielded that responsibility to her lover and her mind fully accepts his/her authority in the matter.

Let's remember, a woman's subconscious mind doesn't usually care who tells it to begin orgasming, it can be her own mind giving the order or it can be her lover's. As a woman you just have to be in the right frame of mind to let it happen.

For 3 hours of sex it is very helpful if the man lasts a long time and/or is capable of getting hard frequently and with minimal downtime.

I last an extremely long time, usually for at least the whole 3 hours. I also have a thick penis which of course is a help.

Incidentally if someone is looking for an easy to find penis desensitizer cream, over the counter hemorrhoid cream under the tip of the penis can work well. I would urge the man to test it out on himself before being with a woman as if too much is used he might not even feel the stimulation enough to get hard! The man needs to know just what the right amount to use is and chances are it's a small amount.

I wanted to note that the dominant sexual position discussed in this book works best when the woman is no more than somewhat overweight.

Here are specifics of what we'd do in our 3 (or more) hour playtime.

1. When you enter my (our) place, you will take off your shoes and go kneel on the thick padding next to my bed (or other agreed upon spot like a chair or couch). Unless told otherwise, your eyes will be looking at where my midsection would be when I sit down in front of you. You will wait for me there (unless of course I'm already there.)

2. I will come over and sit in front of you (assuming I'm not already there.) I may or may not have clothes on. You'll then put your hands on my upper legs, massaging my legs with anticipation. Keep your hands high up on my legs, massaging my legs but you may not touch my penis until allowed to.

3. I will kiss you, touch you, play with you, talk to you and undress you as you kneel in front of me. At some point I may tell you to stand up and take the rest of your clothes off.

4. You will partially or fully undress me when I tell you to. When you pull my pants and underwear down, you know what will pop out!

5. I will then let you suck on my penis. You will first likely have to beg for it though. Also, remember to always play with my testicles while you suck...always!

Rule: Never let any of my penis' ooze go to waste. You know good it tastes! Beg me to let you check for ooze often! Keep sucking my ooze down until I tell you to stop.

6. Soon I will reach down and play with your exposed, vulnerable breasts as you suck on my penis.

7. At some point I may tell you to stop sucking my penis. If so I will then tie your hands securely together.

8. I may tell you to suck on my penis again or we will go straight to the following:

I will sit further back on the bed (or couch/chair) and you will lay stomach down across my lap. I will give you a nice sensual spanking, playing with your body as I do.

I will then tell you to get up and we will go to the bed (if we're not already there.) I will set the bed up so I am sitting with my back against the headboard of the bed and you are laying in front of me face-down on cushions with your head positioned so you can easily suck on my penis and play with my scrotum using your tied-together hands. If I do that though I will make sure there is enough slack in the rope for your hands to still move freely around my penis and scrotum while you suck. If your hands are tied to the middle of the headboard in this manner, I will be sitting on the rope as my butt will be in-between your bound hands and the headboard that your hands are tied to.

9. I'll also put a roughly 4' x 3' (though it can be larger) sheet of strong plastic under your upper body to keep the massage lotion or oil from going on the bed covers. (More on this massage very soon!)

Your breasts will now be positioned, thanks to cushions, so the bottom tips (which will likely be the nipples) of the breasts are just above the bed. As you are lying down and sucking on my penis, I will **generously** lubricate (and keep lubricated,) your breasts with some brand of preferably non-desensitizing lotion or massage oil. The longer the lotion can stay viscous, the better. If warming is necessary (which it most likely will be,) I will warm the lotion/oil up ahead of time or rub it in my hands to warm it up. I will then massage your breasts as you suck on my penis and play with my testicles.

I will continue for a long time to massage your lubricated breasts as you suck on my penis. (This is known as "Extreme Pleasure Breast Massage".) **Remember massagers, <u>always</u> keep you're your hands well lubricated!**

Massager and massagee will quickly notice that the nipples respond with the most pleasure from this type of massage. The massager will find that massaging his lady's breast's large fleshy area first for a while will be quite pleasurable to his slave but it is still not near as pleasurable as briskly massaging her nipples with a circular twisting motion that lets the fingers slide firmly over the nipple, not actually twisting it.

I will first make my lady beg to have her nipples massaged using this Extreme Pleasure Breast Massage technique. My lady has no more than 30 seconds to start her orgasm when I first start giving her Extreme Pleasure Breast Massage. Once I start massaging her nipples, she will have to orgasm a lot harder or risk being punished.

Using a yardstick type implement, I can also reach across your back and spank your bottom as you suck. Obviously one should make sure the woman can handle being spanked while sucking. Most can depending on the intensity of the spanking and how hard she's already orgasming. If she can't one phrase stands out "teeth-marks"!

Optional: After doing this massage for some time, you may wish for the lovely lady to be turned over on her back, her hands still tied to the bed. The man can then eat her. The lady should plan on providing her man with a lot of pussy juice. Should she not provide you with enough pussy juice, feel free to turn her over so her bottom is facing up, and give her a good spanking. Then try eating her again. (Before playing it is important that the lady keep her pussy clean and fresh.) After you've had your fill of her pussy juice, both of you can go back to the original position mentioned in this section or move on to #10.

10. At some point, I may also tie each foot to its corresponding corner of the bed. Instead I may tie your feet securely together and then tie them to the middle of the bed frame at the foot of the bed. Don't worry guys, the placement of a woman's vagina on her body while she's laying on her stomach is such that you still most likely will have easy access even with her legs closed. (However this could be a problem depending on how overweight she and/or he is.)

11. At some point I will order you to stop sucking by saying "head up". I may then get up and give you another spanking as you lay tied down, just for good measure. If you've been a good girl and are getting a lot of pleasure from all this, and if you beg for it, I will put a special vibrator (or two) inside and/or on you and set it up so it stays in place. (Tight underwear and white first aid fabric tape often work best where there are pubic hairs in the area.) I will then return to my original position on the bed and you will continue sucking me and I will also continue giving you Extreme Pleasure Breast Massage (which I promise you'll enjoy immensely!) I will continue to periodically spank you with a yardstick type implement as described earlier.

12. After a while, I will tell you to stop sucking. I'll then clean the lotion, oil, hair conditioner off your breasts with a small towel(s) and remove the small plastic sheet that caught lotion that came off your breasts and my hands. I'll also remove the cushions from under you that kept your breasts literally an inch above the bed. You are now comfortably laying face down on the bed but now without the cushions and plastic under you. You still however are tied down to the bed as you lie on your stomach. (You may wish to put a clean towel under her breasts if they are still a bit oily from the massage.) I will remove any vibrators on and/or in you, as well as whatever was holding them in place. You will be completely naked, tied down, vulnerable and ready to be taken.

13. I will come back in front of you and order you to suck on my penis again. After it is hard, I will dry it off (it must be completely dry for the condom to stay on) and put a condom on it. I will then lay on top of you, stomach down, and enter you with my thick penis.

14. As I take you, you will orgasm for as long as I order you to and orgasm as hard as I order you to. You are required, as part of the orgasm on demand training, to start orgasming within 5 seconds of me entering you. Believe me, it is much easier than it may sound. You will need to ask for permission to start orgasming though! As long as you start asking for permission within 5 seconds of me entering you, you are doing fine. Of course you will need permission to stop your orgasm also! There is the possibility that at some point I will order you to stop your orgasm during our lengthy playtime (or obviously you may have to do that due to unexpected events like the kids coming home early.) If you can however, you are welcome to keep orgasming, even though direct sexual stimulation has temporarily stopped. Once direct sexual stimulation of your breasts and your vagina restarts, you'll of course have to re-start your orgasm once again (assuming it had stopped,) and within 5 seconds as always. (Many of the ladies I have trained will continue orgasming for minutes after physical sexual stimulation has stopped.)

15. As I take you, you will orgasm for as long as I order you to and orgasm as hard as I order you to. Believe me young lady, I require long, hard orgasms from you.

16. As you know I am taking you while both of us are on our stomachs. My stomach of course is on your back. This is far and away the main position I will take you in for the entire time I take you. I may also take you doggie style depending on how overweight she is. There will however not be an emphasis on multiple sex positions during our playtime.

RULE: while I'm playing with you, if you are lying on your stomach and if I ever say "elbows" you are to raise your chest enough so that the tips of your lovely breasts are just above the bed, thus making it easier for me to play with your breasts by sliding one or more of my hands under your chest as I am taking you.

(I think you'll find that my stomach on your back position to be a very good one. Depending on how heavy and/or tall the guy is, you won't have any trouble breathing as my weight is well distributed over your bone-protected pelvis. You won't have to deal with my breathing on your face or you being pounded against the headboard like in the missionary position. Also I can hold you tightly as I take you and easily talk to you as my mouth can be right by your ear.

17. At some point I will slide one or both of my arms under your underarm(s) and put my hands on or around your hands. I can now securely hold you down with my hands. You can now reach my hands (as they are on your wrist, forearms or hands) and kiss them should that be our desire.

18. Sometimes while I am taking you like this, I will spank you. This is accomplished best by me holding myself up with one hand/arm while I am in you and then spanking you with a paddle or the like with the other hand.

19. Often I will hold you down while I take you. I will order you to struggle FROM THE WAIST UP to get free as I am holding you down and taking you at the same time. We will do this one or more times during our long playtime.

20. Sometimes I will take you faster than other times. You will get even more pleasure from this as most any woman would.

21. Sometimes I will thrust into you as deep and hard as I can. You will get even more pleasure from this as most any woman would.

22. This is an excellent sex position for a lady to be taken anally. Perhaps she should have her anus lubed in the beginning when she is originally laid in place incase her man decides to take her anally.

RULE: Remember, the man must always wear a condom when taking her anally and he **can not** re-enter her vagina unless his pubic area has been thoroughly cleaned. A bladder infection is just one of the problems she can have if one doesn't abide by this essential safety tip.

Remember, if something is hurting young lady, you need to tell your man immediately so he can stop.

Well so there are the sexy details of how to play for 3 (or more) hours! Have fun!

Anal stimulation runs the particular risk of spread of disease and all anal activity/penetration requires a high degree of sanitation, before, during and afterward.

Make sure fingernails are well trimmed before using them on a body.

Book #5 – The PS-Spot Orgasm: Don't Wait Any Longer For This Kind of Pleasure

Michelle Tallia

Copyright (C) 2014.

<u>PS-spot.com</u>

It took three tries but it finally happened, my first PS-Spot orgasm, and I want a lot more.

— Jennifer Wilkie, Coopertown, TN

-

When my boyfriend told me about the PS-spot orgasm I didn't believe it but after some research I agreed to give it a try. It hasn't changed my life but it is nice.

— Emma Freedman, Glenwood, AR

-

It finally got me to enjoy anal sex. I'm grateful for that.

— Sara Jones, Davenport, WA

-

My husband's magic fingers have given me a lot of PS-spot orgasms.

Gina K., Galveston, Texas

-

"My husband found my PS-spot and I orgasmed so hard I passed out."

— Molly Sanders, Winston-Salem, NC

Many women know what Perineal Massage is. Women often do this (or have it done to them) to lessen the physical trauma of pushing their babies out of their vagina. Perineal massage involves massaging the perineum (the area located between the anus and the vagina.) This practice is most often done during the final weeks of pregnancy. It protects against tears to the perineal during childbirth.

This book however is about a different perineal related activity.

Learning how to stimulate the female Perineal Sponge (or *PS-Spot* as it's often called) could provide an amazing treat for everybody involved. The PS-Spot can extend an orgasm, make orgasms happen quicker, make them more intense and/or create an orgasm on its own.

The PS-Spot is an often overlooked part of the female sexual anatomy and definitely worth investigating. If you're a man, knowing how to stimulate it (or even knowing of its existence) can really impress a woman. If you're a woman, as you have one, congratulations! Now let's put it to work.

Connected to the truly amazing clitoris is a network of nerves and blood vessels that branch into various clitoral structures. These include the spongy erectile bodies: *the Clitoral Bulbs, the Urethral Sponge and the Perineal Sponge.* The woman's spongy erectile bodies aid intercourse by absorbing her blood like a sponge thus increasing their size and pushing on the vagina walls to make her vagina a tighter fit for the penis. (If one or more of a woman's spongy erectile bodies aren't working properly, it may be noticeable in intercourse as her vagina might not be as tight a fit as expected. This however is not thought to be a wide-spread problem.)

The Perineal Sponge (PS-Spot) is found in the lower genital area of women. Via a wealth of nerves, it's connected to the clitoris. It lies a little (½ to 1½ inches) beneath the perineum (the area between the vaginal and the anus.)

Internally the shaft of the clitoral system divides into two 'legs' that curve downward and look somewhat like a wishbone. These are called "crura", the Latin word for legs. You cannot see or feel these 'legs' but the perineal sponge is connected to the clitoral system largely by these. Mainly because of this connection the *Urethral Sponge* and the *Perineal Sponge* can provide sexual pleasure. (The urethral sponge (the U-spot) is discussed a bit more in depth later on and the author also has written a book on *U-spot sexual pleasure*.)

Both males and females have a *Perineal*. In males it's located where the penis starts (*which is located above the scrotum and called the "bulb of the penis"*) and the anus. In females, it's found between the vagina and anus, roughly 1.25 centimeters from the anus if you start your measurement from the vagina. (That figure can vary.)

As both sexes become sexually aroused, our bodies create substances that cause blood to rush to the genitals, where the blood expands specialized erectile tissue called "bulbs". Men have a single bulb (the bulb of the penis) and women have two bulbs beneath the inner lips of her vagina. If unaroused, normally you can't see or feel the bulbs, but as you're aroused they expand and the genitals become puffed out, creating the female clitoral erection and of course the male erection.

The perineal sponge is internal and often positioned an even distance between the vagina and anus. It's just beneath the perineum. As already noted the perineal sponge (the PS-spot) consists of female erectile tissue. When a woman is sexually stimulated, it fills with blood and becomes enlarged just as a man's penis and a woman's clitoris does during arousal. As it becomes swollen with blood, it compressing the outer third of the vagina creating a tighter fit and thus additional stimulation for the penis. (The *Urethral Sponge* does the same but at a different location of the vagina.)

The PS-spot can also be stimulated through the anus. If you're a fan of anal sex then it's suggested you make a particular effort to stimulate PS-spot during anal sex. Some or more women who orgasm during anal sex may be doing so largely from having their perineal sponge stimulated. These orgasms may be accompanied with ejaculation and may feel similar to orgasms from G-spot stimulation.

A description of the PS-spot comes from sexuality educator Ashley Manta. "If you take your tongue and feel the skin on the roof of your mouth, right behind your {front} teeth, that's what the {stimulated} perineal sponge feels like. It's a little firm, with ridges."

One way to look at it is that if a women is sitting, she has the G-spot on the roof (top) of her vaginal canal and the PS-spot on the floor (bottom) of her vaginal canal.

Note that the PS-Spot is not the same as the "P-Spot" as the P-spot is short for "Prostate Spot" and thus obviously associated only with men, (where the PS-Spot is associated only with women.)

It has been reported that some Tantric sex followers refer to the PS-Spot as the "Cali spot".

How to Stimulate the Perineal Sponge and
Have a PS-Spot Orgasm

The PS-spot is innately erogenous tissue with a large number of nerve endings. It can be stimulated via the vagina or via the rectum (anus), or by stimulating it using both orifices at the same time.

A number of methods can be incorporated to achieve (or at least attempt to achieve) your PS-spot orgasm. You can use fingers (make sure to trim those finger nails down), a variety of toys, particularly curved end vibrating toys, non-vibrating curved end toys, a penis, or a combination. The PS-spot may also be sensitive to massage/pressure when applied directly to the outer perineum (the skin between the vagina and anus.)

Most often however the woman has to first be sexually excited to get the desired impact from PS-spot stimulation. In other words first get aroused then start the PS-spot stimulation.

PS-spot stimulation can be accomplished by masturbation or by a lover.

▶ There's an online videoclip showing how to find and stimulate the PS-Spot at www.orgasmarts.com/ps-spot (Orgasm Arts). Please note, it shows naked female genitalia, so only look at it in private. The writer and publisher of this book are not associated with this graphic but very informative videoclip.

Often it's best to simultaneously stimulate the PS-spot from both top and bottom by using well manicured, very clean fingers and/or toys in both her anus and vagina at the same time.

For simplicity, let's start with accessing the PS-spot by only using one of those entrances at a time.

1) Often, *(1)* well manicured, very clean fingers, or *(2)* very clean curved-tip toys, are best for attaining sexual pleasure from the perineal sponge, (the PS-spot). This is compared to intercourse, though many women get PS-spot orgasms from intercourse.

2) Many of the same suggestions for stimulating the G-spot holds true for stimulating the PS-spot, except the PS-Spot typically is not as far into the vagina.

To look for the G-spot, after she's sexually aroused, insert one or two fingers in the vagina with your palm facing her vagina. Gently bend your fingers up towards her head so that they stroke the front wall (thus the upper wall if she's lying on her back) of her vagina. You may feel a raised spot or series of ridges, or nothing in particular. The woman may find this extremely pleasurable, or may have an urge to urinate, or both. Stroking this area with varying degrees of pressure will most likely tell the woman if she's got a G-spot or not.

To find the PS-spot using this type of method, remember that it's on the opposite part of her vagina so the hand doing the stimulating/searching likely will need to turn 180 degrees. Also it is only ½ to 1½ inches in to the vagina versus 2-3 inches in to the vagina as are most G-spots.

The G-Spot, or Grafenberg Spot is named after its discoverer, a German gynecologist called Ernst Grafenberg. It's defined as a bean-shaped area of the vagina that when stimulated, can lead to strong sexual arousal, powerful orgasms and female ejaculation. It's sometimes referred to as the *Goddess Spot*. 1940s research into the female orgasm led to the discovery that the female's urethral tube, which lies on top of the vagina, is surrounded by erectile tissue similar to that found in the male penis. When the female becomes sexually aroused, this tissue swells. In the G-spot zone this expansion results in a small protrusion through the vaginal wall that protrudes into the vaginal canal. It's this raised patch that is, according to Grafenberg, "a primary erotic zone, perhaps more important than the clitoris." {That is something that has been proven to be incorrect.} He stated that its significance was lost when the 'missionary position' became a dominant feature of human sexual behavior as there are other sexual positions that are more efficient at stimulating this erogenous zone (the G-spot.)

The term "G-spot" was not used by Grafenberg himself, he called it "an erotic zone", which actually is a better description of it. Unfortunately, the modern use of "G-spot" as a popular term has led to some misunderstandings. Some women mistakenly believe that there is a 'magic sexual pleasure button' that can be activated at any time to get great pleasure. The truth is that the G-spot is a sexually sensitive patch in the vaginal wall that protrudes slightly only when the glands surrounding the urethral tube have become swollen (mainly the *urethral sponge*). Importantly, the woman needs to be significantly sexually stimulated first to get it to do that.

For a while the sexual establishment denied the existence of such a thing. Sexual politics had reared its ugly head. (Remember this was in the 1940s and 50s. Women back then still weren't expected to get great pleasure from sex and many questioned whether a vaginal orgasm was even possible. They tended to believe a clitoral orgasm was possible though.)

There have been reports of women undergoing 'G-spot enhancement'. This involves injecting collagen into the G-spot zone to enlarge it (thus pushing it further into the vagina so it interacts with the thrusting penis more.) According to one source, "One of the latest procedures to catch on is *G-spot injection*. The idea is that this will increase its sensitivity and give you better orgasms."

The fact is that a large number of women are getting enhanced sexual pleasure and/or orgasms by stimulating the area where the G-spot is suppose to be but there remains a major controversy as to whether the G-spot even exists. The writer of this book assumes the G-spot exists but has no conclusive proof.

Finding Your G-spot

Here is one of the suggested ways to find your *G-spot*. Make sure you're quite sexually aroused. Insert one or two fingers (a vibrating curved tip toy may work better) two inches into the vagina and starting at the top of the vagina, exert the necessary force, or vibrating force, at the 12 o-clock position. If your G-spot doesn't make its presence known, try repeating this process *further in* another third of an inch, then another third of an inch and then to play it safe another third of an inch and maybe another third. If it hasn't made its presence felt yet, do the same procedure, but starting from two inches in *at the 12:30 position* and if necessary then again at the 1:00 position. If the G-spot remains hidden try this procedure in the 11:30 position and the 11:00 o'clock position. There are reports of women finding their G-spots in the 10:00, 10:30, 1:30 and 2:00 position. Again you want to start testing from two inches into the vagina (or maybe start at 1½ inches to play it safe) and then further and further into your vagina. Most G-spots, if they're found, are found 2-3 inches in from the front of the vagina, but yours might be located outside those parameters. Please note that you may be one of the hundreds of millions of women that don't have a G-spot and there remains some doubt in academic circles as to whether it really even exists. Assuming it exists, as previously noted, it's located in the vicinity of the urethral sponge, not the perineal sponge.)

In 2011, researcher Adam Ostrzenski claimed to have found the first evidence of G-spot anatomical structures by dissecting a cadaver in Poland. Between the fifth and sixth layer of the vaginal wall, there were grape-like clusters Ostrzenski believed were erectile tissue that would have functioned as a G-spot {or stimulated it.} The research was published in *The Journal of Sexual Medicine* in 2012. Critics of Ostrzenski's claim note that he provided no evidence that his sample consisted of nerve endings with structures that played a role in arousal, or that they would be in one specific area. Ostrzenski said that part of the reason he didn't detail a precise type of tissue and how it works is because of Polish regulations that govern dissection of fresh cadavers. It prevented him from taking samples for histological testing. He said that he was not suggesting that the G-spot he reported would be found in the same place, or have the same effect, for every woman.*

*(Healy, Melissa (April 25, 2012). "Doctor says he's found the actual G spot".) (Taken from http://en.wikipedia.org/wiki/G-spot).

Locating and/or Stimulating Your PS-Spot via the Vagina

If a woman is lying on her back, the *back (posterior)* wall of the vagina is the part of her vagina that is closest to the bed, and the *lower* part of her vagina is the part of her vagina that's closest to the vagina's entrance.

As the PS-spot is erectile tissue, typically the woman needs to be turned on sexually for it to be most significantly activated (filled with blood and thus 'erect'.) By activated I mean getting firmer to the touch. This can be accomplished in the usual manner, through breast stimulation, clitoral stimulation or even kissing depending on how quickly and easily she gets sexually stimulated. In other words in many cases it doesn't work as well to start playing with her PS-spot if she isn't already turned on.

When only using the vagina for PS-spot stimulation, (versus using both the vagina and anus simultaneously,) the PS-spot can be accessed via the *lower back* wall of the vagina. It's between ½ to 1½ inches into the vagina. Your *well manicured, very clean* finger or toy enters the vagina and pushes down toward the anus. Start by pushing down only a half inch in, then a little further in until she feels the stimulation. (Typically it's not more than 1½ inches into the vagina.) You flick/move your finger in a manner that gives her the most pleasure. If you're using a toy perhaps sliding it back and forth a bit will do the trick, particularly if it's a vibrating toy. However please note, many women simply don't have a PS-spot, or at least one at that time of her life.

2) If a woman wants to try to stimulate her perineal sponge during intercourse, either with a penis or dildo, she should position herself in a manner that directs the phallic implement of choice toward the back (thus bottom if she's laying on her back,) wall of the vagina. Three recommended sexual positions are:

- The missionary position
- The woman-on-top position
- Seated and facing each other.

You want to do the opposite of what works best for targeting the G-spot. For instance doggy style vaginal intercourse is a good G-spot sex position but not as good for the PS-spot.

Locating and/or Stimulating Your PS-Spot via the Anus

The rectum lies against the sacrum (lower backbone) in a gentle curve down to the anal opening which as you know is penetrated during anal sex. The front (anterior) wall of the rectum and rear wall of the vagina, and the thin layer of tissue between them, are together called the *rectovaginal septum* (or wall).

Anally the perineal sponge can be accessed via the front wall of the rectum. (If a woman is lying on her back, the *front wall* of the rectum is that which is closest to her vagina.)

Use a *well manicured, very clean finger* (and remember to keep anything that has touched her anus, away from her vagina. That's important!)

► There's an online videoclip showing how to find and stimulate the PS-Spot at www.orgasmarts.com/ps-spot (Orgasm Arts). Please note, it shows naked female genitalia, so only look at it in private. The writer and publisher of this book are not associated with this graphic but very informative videoclip.

As the man's prostate is stimulated from being taken anally (as that's his *P-spot*), conversely a woman's PS-spot can be stimulated from being taken anally.

A reason the G-spot feels good when touched is because it stimulates the clitoris from the clitoris' underside. The clitoris isn't just what you see on the outside. It actually goes roughly a couple inches inside of a woman.

The PS-spot is located closer to the rectum than the G-spot, though further from the clitoris. (but remember the PS-spot is connected to the powerful clitoral system via the clitoris' crura.)

1) When testing to see if a woman has a PS-spot, it could be best to first explore for, and/or stimulate the potential PS-spot location with a thinner sex toy, or normal size finger. (Trim the finger nail!!!) Remember its located ½ to 1½ inches in from the vagina's entrance. A wider sex toy, or a penis, should the receiver not be used to it, could cause physical anxiety and/or trauma that takes away from the PS-spot sexual enhancement experience.

2) Generally speaking, fingers or curved-tip toys are best for applying pressure on the perineal sponge, whether insertion is occurring via the vagina or via the anus. In many cases though, simple insertion by a penis *into the anus* versus the vagina can have more success stimulating the PS-spot than simple insertion by a penis into the vagina. Chances are good that if a woman orgasms from anal sex alone, at least part of that is from PS-spot stimulation.

As previously noted the PS-spot is located between the rectum and vagina so when insertion of a toy or phallus is occurring in the anus, the emphasis/pressure should be on the part the rectum closest to the vagina.

Locating and/or Stimulating Your PS-Spot by Utilizing the Anus and Vagina at the Same Time.

This is the preferred way to search for and activate her PS-spot, but remember anything that touches the anus cannot touch the vagina!

1) The woman should be sexually excited so the erectile tissue, which includes the perineal sponge, has filled or is filling with blood. This makes the PS-spot easier to find and more sensitive.
2) Use plenty of lubricant.
3) Use a *well manicured, very clean finger/thumb to* enter her vagina and another finger/thumb to enter her anus at the same time.
4) Massage, rub and/or vibrate the PS-spot (which is between the two openings) simultaneously from insertion into both the top and bottom 'holes'. The PS-spot is located only ½ to 1½ inches in from their entrances.
5) Just because she didn't orgasm from it this time or not get a great deal of pleasure doesn't mean she won't when you do it again in the future.

While having intercourse, one of the parties can stimulate the PS-spot through the unoccupied opening, or even the outside of the *Perineal* (which is the skin between the vagina and anus.)

The Perineal Sponge may respond to pressure from the outside of the perineal body.

The perineal sponge may respond to pressure from outside the body too, though this could depend on how much fat and muscle is in between it and your skin. Try a vibrator that you would normally use on your clitoris and press and move it against the skin that is located equidistant between the vagina and anus. Chances are good pushing up will help. With experimentation you can determine the best way to stimulate the PS-spot this way, if your PS-spot can even can be stimulated this way.

Stimulating the Urethral Sponge

The perineal sponge is not the same as the urethral sponge. Like the perineal sponge the urethral sponge is a spongy cushion of erectile tissue found in the lower genital area of women. It sits against both the pubic bone and vaginal wall and surrounds the urethra. Its job however is much the same as the perineal sponge. With sexual stimulation, it engorges itself with blood and makes a tighter more pleasurable fit for the penis. It is however closer to the clitoris.

The G-spot is located in the urethral sponge and one theory is that as the urethral sponge engorges itself with blood from sexual excitement, it pushes down on the G-spot area which more fully activates the G-spot's clitoral nerve connection, giving the woman sexual pleasure.

The urethral sponge provides women with the "U-spot". The U-spot can be located in different parts of the urethral sponge; its size can vary from woman to woman. (Unfortunately many women don't have a pleasurable U-spot to start out with.) The U-spot isn't the same as the G-spot but the G-spot can be located in the often bigger U-Spot.

The urethral sponge encompasses sensitive nerve endings connected to the clitoris. It can be stimulated through the front wall of the vagina. Some women experience intense pleasure from stimulation of the urethral sponge (U-spot) while others find the sensation irritating. The urethral sponge surrounds clitoral nerves, and since the two are so closely interconnected, stimulation of the clitoris may stimulate the nerve endings of the urethral sponge and vice versa. Some women get U-spot pleasure from the rear-entry position of *vaginal intercourse* (whether she's laying on her stomach or on her hands and knees) as the penis is often angled slightly downward and can stimulate the front wall of the vagina, and in turn the urethral sponge.

If you have a pleasurable U-spot you want to get to know it better as there is documented evidence of women getting earth-shattering orgasms from it as women have with the PS-spot.

Conclusion

Women, enhance your sexual pleasure with a part of your body you already have and likely are not even using!

Is the PS-Spot also one of your hot spots? I certainly hope so and for many people it is. (Incidentally if the G-spot isn't a hotspot for you, don't assume the PS-Spot won't be also, as actually often it is.) Unfortunately there's no guarantee that optimal utilization of any sexual part of your body will make you scream like a ban chi. The important thing is that you explored an erroneous zone in your body (and there are others) to make sure you can be all you can be.

▶ There's an online videoclip showing how to find and stimulate the PS-Spot at www.orgasmarts.com/ps-spot (Orgasm Arts). Please note, it shows naked female genitalia, so only look at it in private. The writer and publisher of this book are not associated with this graphic but very informative videoclip.

Guys, an easy, cheap way to delay ejaculation is: anti-hemorrhoidal and anesthetic ointments. I know a man who used NUPERCAINAL for that purpose. It's an over-the-counter medicine and readily available at many drug stores. I suggest however that you only put *very little* on as it's very potent. You want to mainly put it on the underside of the tip of the penis. It will be absorbed by the skin after a while. *Guys you'll have to test it yourself to see what the best amount for your use is because if you put too much on (which is easy to do) you might not feel her stroking you in an attempt to make you hard.* Please note this disclaimer. I do not know if there are any side effects to its use and though I don't know of anybody having a problem with it, it's possible. Contact a physician before using it.

The End